Exercise *Without* Movement

Exercise Without Movement

Manual One

As Taught by
Sri Swami Rama
of the Himalayas

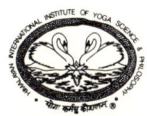

The Himalayan International Institute
of Yoga Science and Philosophy of the U.S.A.
Honesdale, Pennsylvania

Illustrations: Michael Smith
Photographs: Dave Gorman,
Model: Doug Bill

© 1984 Swami Rama

The Himalayan International Institute of
Yoga Science and Philosophy of the U.S.A.
RR 1, Box 400
Honesdale, Pennsylvania 18431

All rights reserved. No part of this book may be reproduced in any form or by any means without permission in writing from the publisher. Printed in the United States of America.

Second printing 1986

The paper used in this publication meets the minimun requirements of American National Standard for Information Sciences—Permanence of Paper for Printed Library Materials, ANSI Z39.48-1984. ∞

Library of Congress Cataloging in Publication Data:

Rama, Swami, 1925-
    Exercise without movement.

    (Manual ; 1)
    1. Yoga, Hatha. 2. Stretch (Physiology) 3. Muscle tone. 4. Relaxation. I. Title. II. Series: Manual (Himalayan International Institute of Yoga Science & Philosophy of the USA) ; 1.
RA781.7.R26   1984   613.7′046   84-20500
ISBN 0-89389-089-8

Contents

Foreword—by Swami Ajaya, Ph.D.　　　　　　　ix

Preface　　　　　　　xi

Introduction　　　　　　　3

Part One
　Basic Relaxation　　　　　　　7

Part Two
　Tension/Relaxation Exercise　　　　　　　13

Part Three
　The Boat Pose　　　　　　　33

Part Four
　Ashvini Mudra　　　　　　　37

Part Five
　The Child's Pose　　　　　　　41

Part Six
　Standing Tension/Relaxation　　　　　　　45

Part Seven
　Agni Sara　　　　　　　51

Part Eight
　Shavayatra　　　　　　　57

Part Nine
    Two to One Breathing   65

Appendix I
    Preparations for Practice   71

Appendix II
    Diaphragmatic Breathing   73

Appendix III
    Corpse Pose Relaxation   77

Appendix IV
    Summary at a Glance   81

List of Illustrations

The crocodile pose	8, 81
The corpse pose	10, 58, 76, 81
Right leg tensed	14, 82
Left leg tensed	16, 82
Both legs tensed	18, 82
Right side tensed	20, 83
Left side tensed	22, 83
Right arm tensed	24, 84
Left arm tensed	24, 84
Both arms tensed	28, 84
All limbs tensed	30, 85
The boat pose	34, 85
Ashvini mudra	38, 86
The child's pose	42, 86

Standing against a wall	46, 87
Agni sara	52, 87
Pelvic contraction in agni sara	54
31 points	60
61 points	62, 88
Sitting on a chair	66, 88
The easy pose	68, 88
The auspicious pose	68
The diaphragm	74

Foreword

There are many types of exercises known in both the East and the West. Each has a place in helping to make various aspects of the human organism healthy and vigorous. Aerobic exercises, isometrics, and yogic exercises are each useful in their own way. After considering and experimenting with all such exercises, one is led to the conclusion that they focus primarily on the physical body, strengthening muscles or improving the cardiovascular system, for example. The exercises in this book are unique, for all efforts are first mental, and then the body acts accordingly. Here mind and body are trained together.

When a student learns to do these exercises it leads him to a state of mind in which he is able to control the so-called involuntary system at will. The exercises in this book prevent the occurrence of various psychosomatic disorders that originate from the nervous system, bad breathing habits, or lack of concentration. A dissipated mind is a source of many disorders, but those disorders will be eliminated if one masters the program offered here.

These exercises were carefully designed by Swami Rama, who came to the United States in the early 1970s and participated in extensive research on the voluntary control of internal states at the Menninger Foundation. Swamiji also pioneered in the development of biofeedback as a means for voluntarily controlling internal states. In this book he has brought together in a succinct form some of the most effective methods for mastering mind and body. These exercises have been developed and applied over thousands of years. At first glance they may appear deceptively simple for achieving such remarkable results. But as one goes on practicing and reaches new levels of awareness, he finds that even more subtle mastery of mind and body is attained.

While Swamiji was teaching students, Rolf Sovik, director of the Center for Higher Consciousness in Minneapolis, Minnesota, carefully compiled these exercises. They may be practiced by people of all ages, and through regular practice various aspects of the aging process will be arrested. They will help one to remain strong, youthful, and vigorous, yet calm and serene. I hope that those who read this book will practice these methods systematically so that they can acquire and enjoy health and vitality on all levels of their being.

Swami Ajaya, Ph.D.

Preface

Yoga is a word that has been repeatedly used in the most ancient scriptures of man, the Vedas. It is found in the Yajurveda, and means "to unite" or "to join." Eventually we must all unite our individual souls with the cosmic One. To do this we must systematically understand our body, breath, senses, mind, and the Center of consciousness within, from which consciousness flows in various degrees and grades. Once you have known yourself, you have known the Self of all, and you comprehend the mysteries of life here and hereafter.

To make such a journey, however, we must start from the beginning. There are many kinds of physical exercises in yoga; these have varying effects on mind and body. One collection of exercises is considered to be the most subtle. These exercises are practiced internally, without movement, and have a profound effect. They will help you understand your mind and its relationship with the breath and physical body.

These exercises lead to mastery over the involuntary nervous system. You will learn how your heart, intestines, and brain function. You can have mastery over all these functions, if you really know the body, breath, senses, and mind to be your instruments. You can and should have control over these instruments. All the functions of personality can serve the final goal of human destiny: liberation, or moksha.

The exercises have many practical benefits, but to reap them, you will have to practice regularly. It is also important to practice in the proper way and never to exceed your capacity in performing the exercises. In electricity, if the current exceeds the capacity of the circuit through which the energy flows, a fuse will blow out. This is also the case with the human nervous system. In the body, the sign of excessive tension is shaking. When the body shakes from tension then the capacity of the nervous system has been exceeded.

With practice a time will come when the discomfort of extreme temperature, the incapacities of aging, and the disruption caused by unexpected emotional turmoil will not affect you. Your body will become free from many diseases like coronary heart disease and others involving the nervous system.

So, may your practice of these exercises progress without interruption. May you practice with full zeal and with full determination. Tell yourself from the very beginning that you will succeed. Don't fall back into old grooves. You can create new grooves that will carry you along on your way. Simply fix a time, and practice at that time each day. You will enjoy these exercises very much.

Exercise *Without* Movement

Introduction

At first thought it may seem incongruous to "exercise" without movement. Normally we associate exercise with physical activity like swimming, jogging, tennis, or walking. Each of these forms of exercise plays a role in maintaining good health. The exercises in this book, however, are yoga practices with benefits far exceeding ordinary muscular movement. In these subtle exercises one vitalizes muscles, respiration, senses, nervous system, and mind.

What is "exercise without movement"? Holding your arm straight out in front of you, you will find that you can alternately tense and relax the biceps muscle while creating very little movement of the arm itself. You are flexing a muscle without moving the body part to which it is attached. When the mind sends the command, one feels the effect in the body, but normally, little more of the process than this is observed. Exercise without movement, however, is a systematic method of exercise that allows the practitioner to travel along the pathways of action, from mind to muscle. The tension/relaxation process is carefully observed, and the health of each link in the process is promoted. Many parts of the body that do not normally receive much exercise are thereby stimulated.

In the beginning of practice some simple discoveries are made. For instance, one finds that activity involving the system of muscles and nerves has two boundaries. The first boundary is the upper limit of tension beyond which the muscle begins to shake. Another boundary is the state of full relaxation, beyond which no more tension can be released. The following exercises lead to both of these boundaries through systematic tension and relaxation. Each exercise focuses on a particular group of muscles, and gradually, through mastery of the exercises, the capacity to tense and relax these muscles is expanded. The student also begins to maintain the correct level of muscle tone for optimum health.

It is very important to learn to discriminate while performing the exercises. If the right leg is to be tensed, then the left leg should be relaxed, and no sympathetic tension need arise in other parts of the body. You will learn to tense one limb so that it can hardly be lifted, while the other limbs remain limp and flexible.

Accompanying the tension/relaxation exercises are a number of other yoga practices. Each is effective in improving the processes of cleansing, nourishing, and vitalizing the human system. It is important to include all the exercises rather than practice some to the exclusion of others.

Through yoga practice, various levels of the human organism and personality are systematically experienced, from the gross elements that constitute the human body, to the subtle-most layers of mind that are illumined by joy and tranquility. These exercises help the student move from the gross to the more subtle. Relaxed self-observation throughout the exercises is the key to enhancing this process.

Before practicing the exercises the student should have a practical knowledge of diaphragmatic breathing and should be familiar with the essential principles of hatha yoga. It is worth repeating, even for experienced students, that hatha yoga practices should begin only after food has been digested, wastes eliminated, and a caring attitude for the body has been cultivated. Appendixes with more information are provided in the back of this manual.

Photographs of all the important postures accompany the descriptions of the exercises. One should study the pictures carefully and try to assume the same posture for individual practice. Careful attention to one's own capacity should also be paid. If muscle tension is introduced gradually, there will be a feeling of strength and confidence, with no shaking or overexertion.

These exercises lead toward the fulfillment of the purpose of hatha yoga. They are the preliminary steps to mastery of the autonomic nervous system. At the same time they prevent many diseases that modern medicine has found difficult to treat and cure. Most importantly, in these exercises one comes to experience the tremendous potential of the mind itself, and one makes a dramatic step inward through the layers of personality toward the Center of mind and consciousness.

The following series of exercises is to be practiced from beginning to end. After the initial learning period, you will find that a span of about thirty to forty-five minutes is sufficient to complete the entire series. Choose a time when you will not be interrupted, and practice regularly each day. These exercises are suitable for both men and women. Students are advised to carefully review Appendix I before commencing their practice.

PART ONE
Basic Relaxation

8 / *Exercise Without Movement*

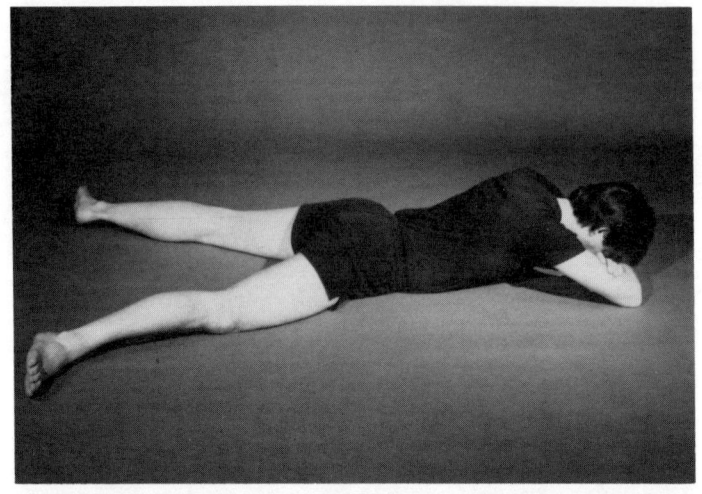

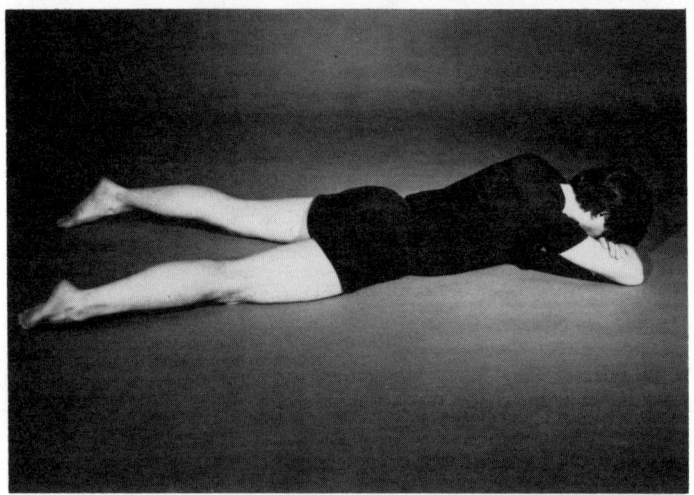

The crocodile pose

ONE
Crocodile Relaxation

Lie on the stomach, placing the legs a comfortable distance apart and pointing the toes in or out, whichever is more comfortable. Fold the arms in front of the body, resting the hands on the biceps. Position the arms so that the chest does not touch the floor, as pictured. Then place the forehead on the forearms.

This posture enables you to establish diaphragmatic breathing (see Appendix II). You may use a cloth beneath the nostrils to keep from inhaling dust. As you lie in the posture, observe your breathing. Let the breath become deep and smooth. While inhaling, feel the abdominal muscles gently press against the floor; while exhaling, feel the abdomen contract. Let the body relax completely.

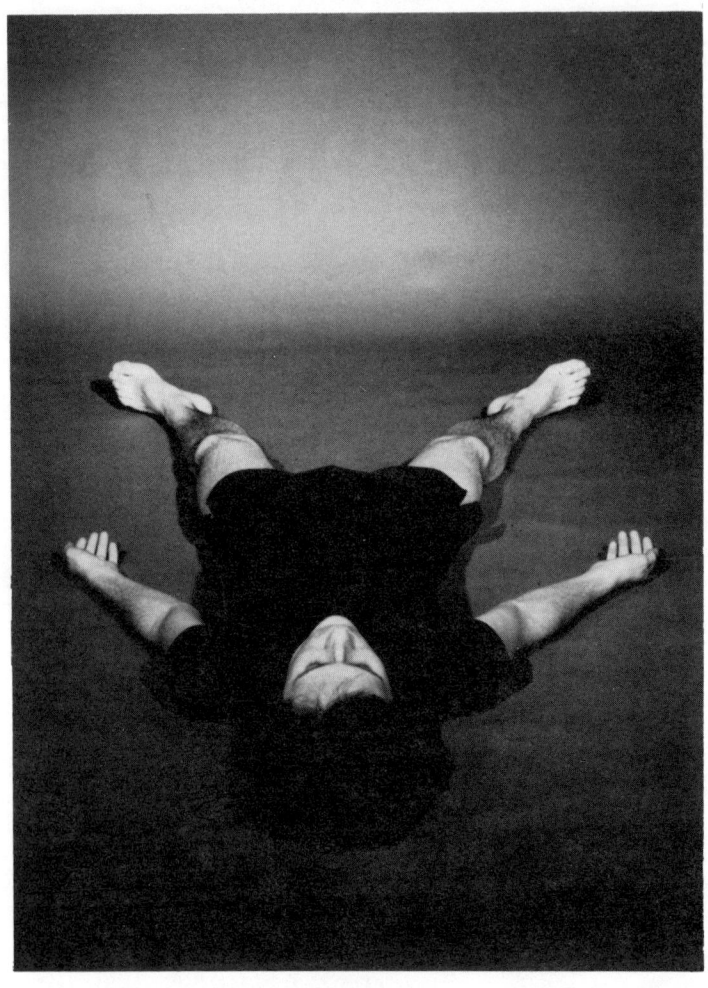

The corpse pose

TWO
Corpse Pose Relaxation

Roll onto your back and again breathe diaphragmatically, exhaling waste and fatigue and inhaling a feeling of vitality. Lie with your spine straight. The arms and legs are a comfortable distance apart, with the palms turned up. You may use a thin cushion under the neck and head.

Relax systematically by moving the body parts gently from side to side and then becoming still. Follow this sequence: right leg, right arm, left leg, left arm, torso, neck, and head. Again, let the body relax completely.

PART TWO
Tension/Relaxation Exercise

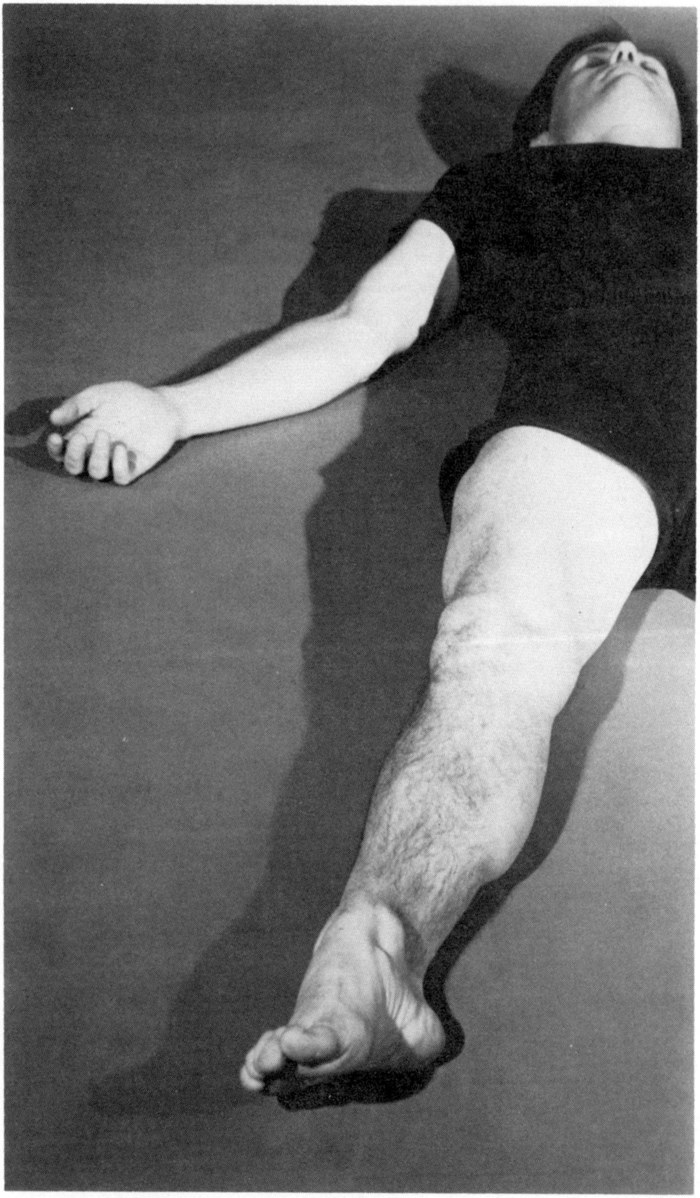

14 / *Exercise Without Movement*

Right leg tensed

ONE
The Legs

Right Leg

Lying in the corpse pose, bring your attention to your right leg. Consciously create tension in the toes, pointing them away from the body. Do not tense any other part of your leg until you have given the conscious command. Now continue the tension upward through the foot, to the ankle joint. The whole foot will point away from the body. Continue the tension to the knee joint, tensing the calf muscles and muscles of the lower thigh. Finally move the tension upward through the entire leg, from the toes to the uppermost muscles of the thigh. If there is shaking, you have tensed too much and gone beyond your capacity. Reduce the tension slightly by relaxing your effort.

Hold the tension briefly. If you observe tension arising in any other part of your body, relax it. Only your right leg is tensed. Continue to breathe deeply and smoothly.

Relax the tension slowly from the toes, in the same order in which you have created tension. Release all the tension, and let the leg roll back to the side.

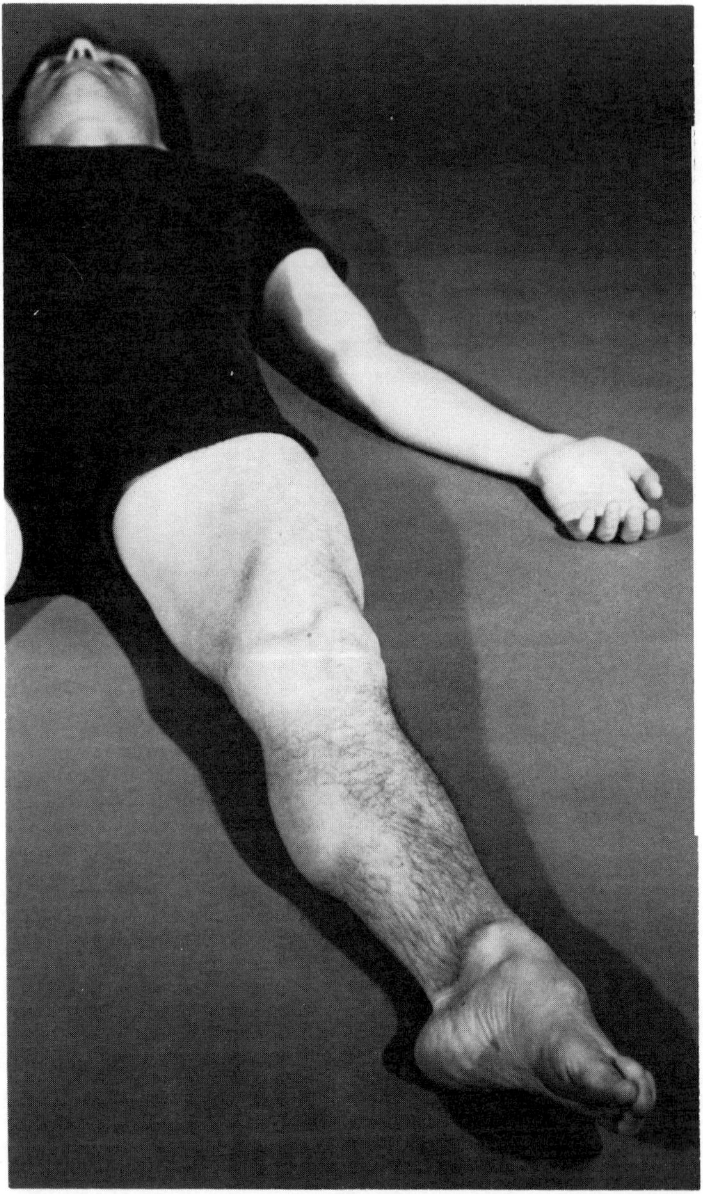

16 / *Exercise Without Movement*

Left leg tensed

Left Leg

Repeat the exercise with the left leg, slowly and systematically. Watch for sympathetic tension in the opposite leg. Note that the tense muscles become very hard, almost "like rock."

Repeat

Do the tension/relaxation a second time on each leg, right leg and then left leg.

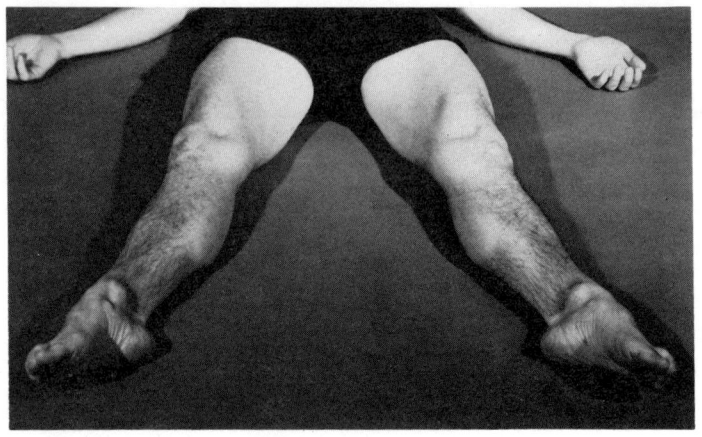

Both legs tensed

Both Legs

Finally perform the tension/relaxation exercise with both legs simultaneously. Do not allow tension in the upper part of the body. Continue to breathe slowly and smoothly throughout.

Repeat

After relaxing, repeat the exercise.

Relaxed Breathing

When you are finished with both legs, relax completely and breathe out and in, two times. In the beginning if you wish to relax a little longer, you may.

Now go on to the next step.

20 / *Exercise Without Movement*

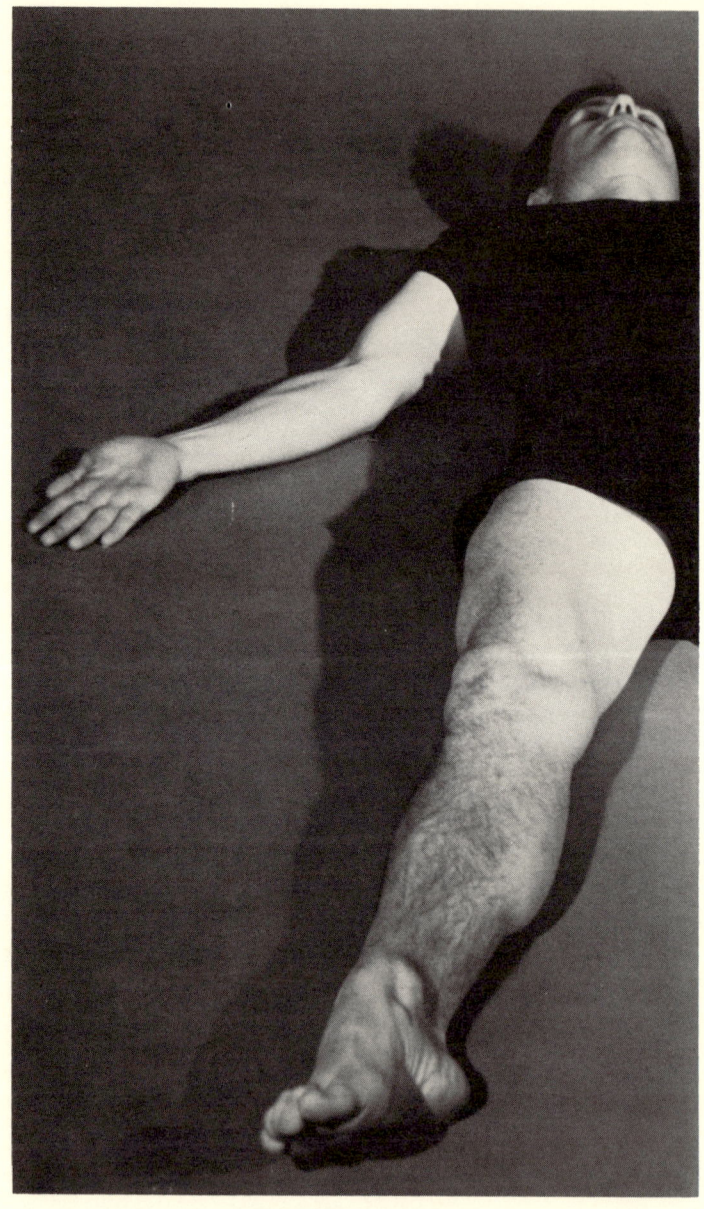

Right side tensed

TWO
Right Side/Left Side

Right Side

Tense the right leg and right arm simultaneously. When tensing the arm, the palm of the hand is open and turned upward with fingers together. The tension moves from the fingertips, through the hand and upward to the muscles of the upper arm. As before, all the tension is under conscious control and the mind moves slowly up the arm. Two feelings are distinct: 1) the fingers (and palm) become straight and stiff, resting on the ground but not pressing it, and 2) the muscle of the upper arm seems to rotate outward as it becomes tense. The arm will feel fully open. As you tense the right leg and right arm simultaneously, move the tension upward slowly from the toes and the fingertips.

Hold the tension, without letting any tension arise in the left half of your body. Your breath remains smooth and deep.

Release the tension systematically, again moving upward from the toes and the fingertips.

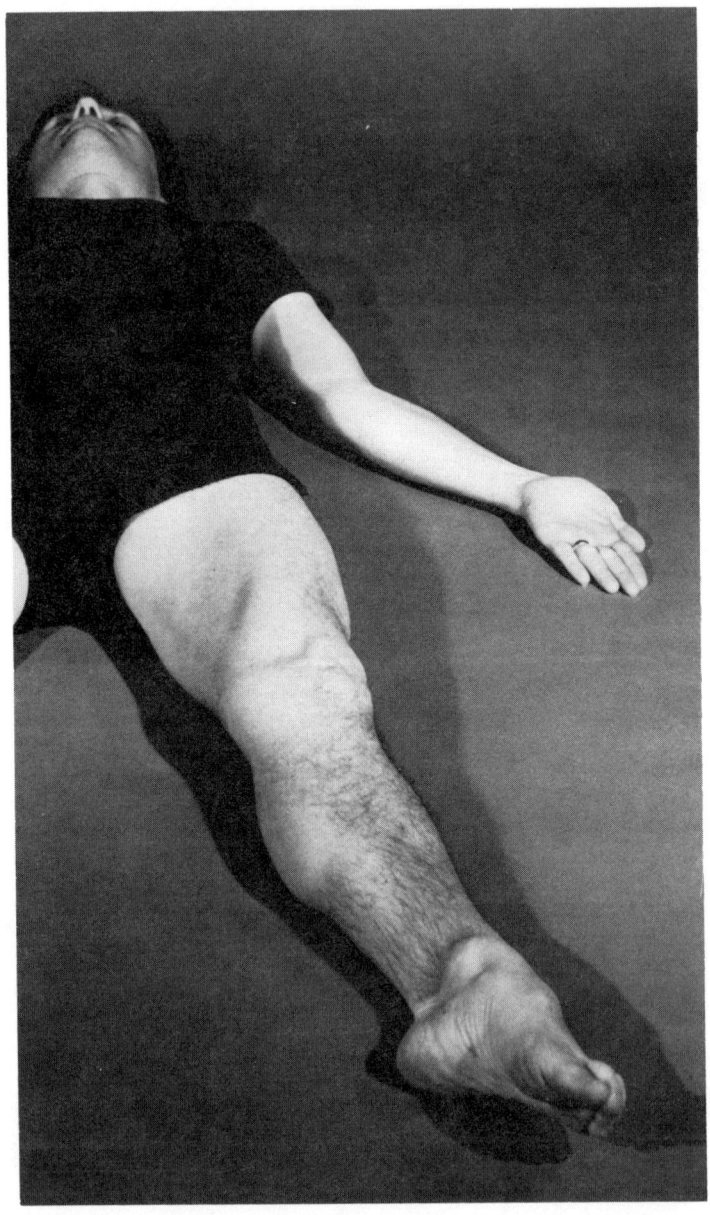

Left side tensed

Left Side

Do the tension/relaxation on the left side of the body. You may notice a difference in capacity or muscular control from one side of the body to the other. These exercises will help you to balance the two sides of your body.

Repeat

Do the tension/relaxation again on each side, right and then left.

Relaxed Breathing

When you have finished, relax completely and breathe out and in, two times.

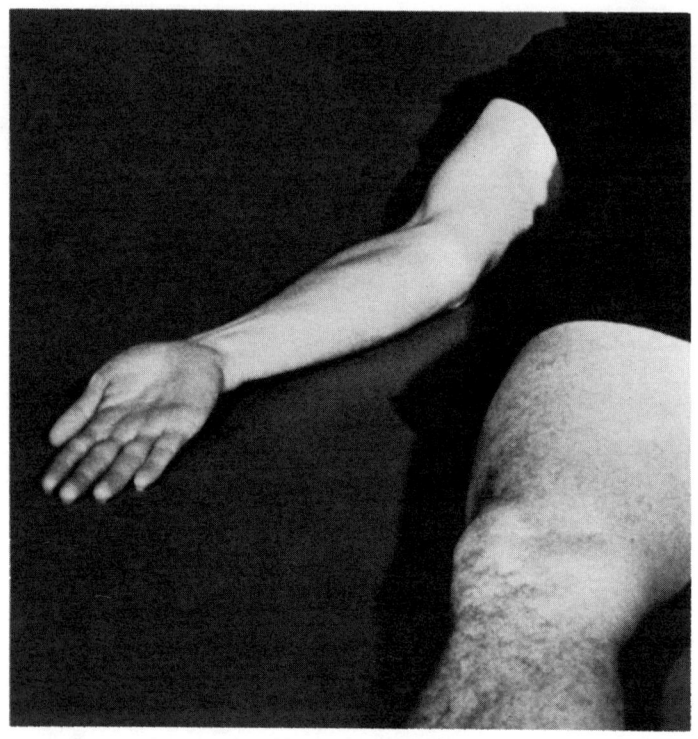

Right arm tensed

THREE
The Arms

Right Arm

Begin by tensing the arm from the fingertips, as described in step two (page 21). Move the tension upward through the fingers, palm, wrist, lower arm, elbow, and upper arm. Do not lift the shoulder.

Hold the tension, observing your capacity.

Relax slowly from the fingertips.

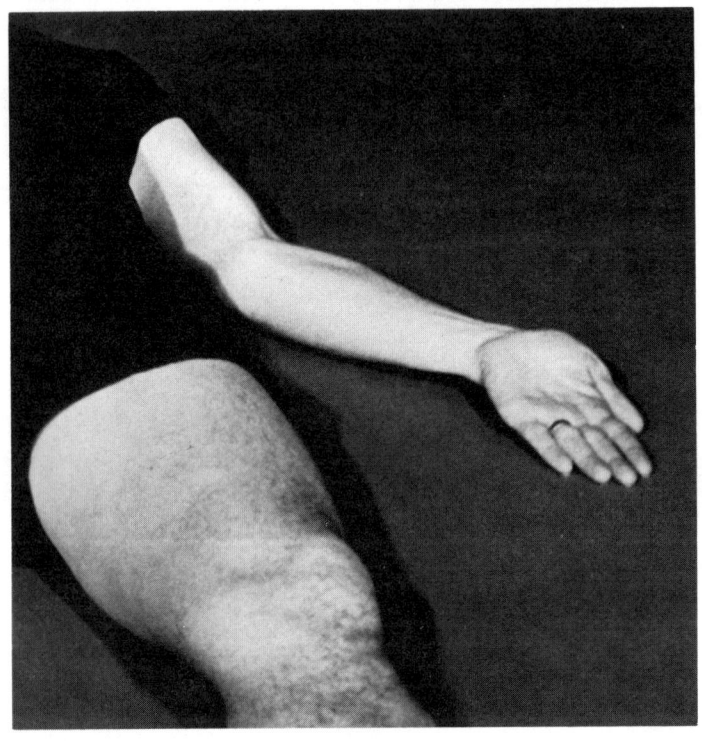

Left arm tensed

Left Arm

Do the exercise with the left arm.

Repeat

Perform the exercise again with each arm, right and then left.

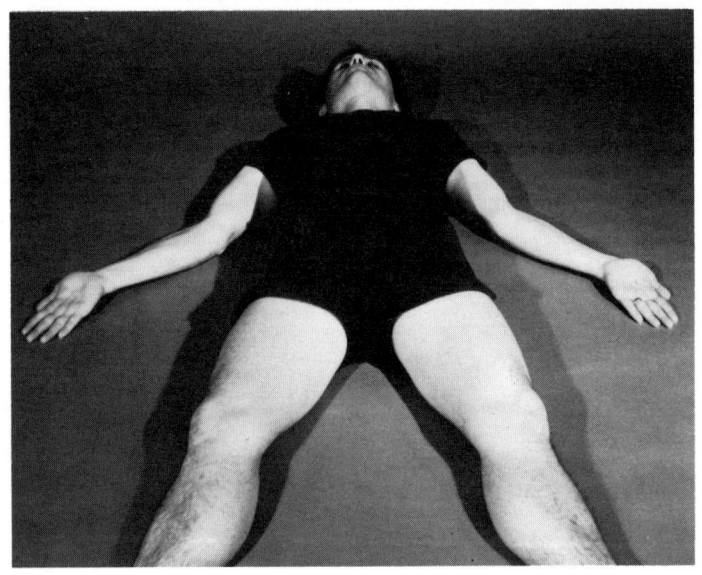

Both arms tensed

Both Arms

Do the tension/relaxation exercise with both arms. Do not allow sympathetic tension in the lower extremities. Continue to breathe slowly and smoothly.

Repeat

Tense both arms again.

Relaxed Breathing

When you have finished, relax completely and breathe out and in, two times.

30 / *Exercise Without Movement*

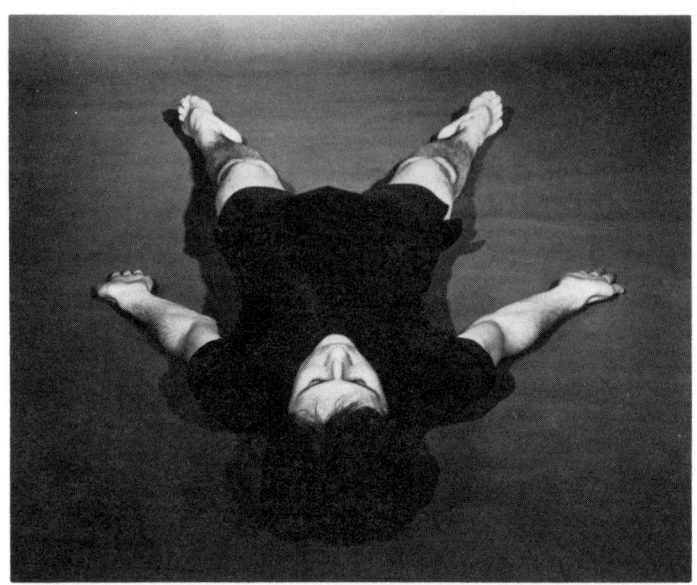

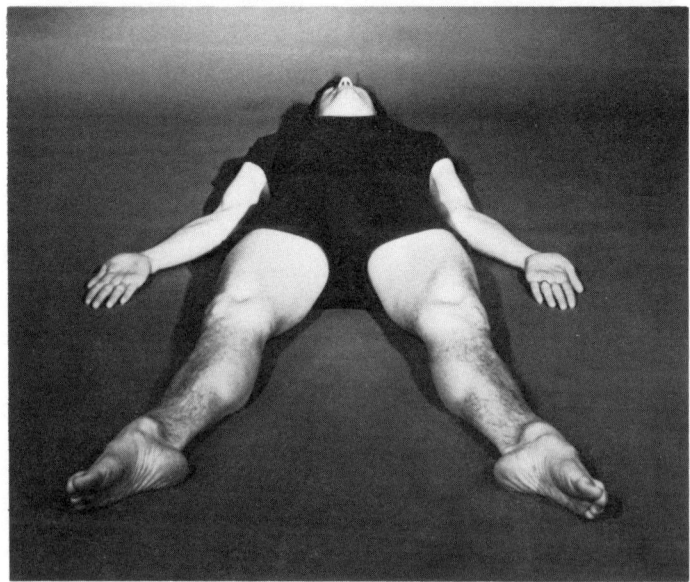

All limbs tensed

FOUR
The Whole Body

All The Limbs

Finally, tense all the limbs simultaneously using the same method you have used in the individual exercises:

    A.   Create the muscular tension systematically from the mind.

    B.   Hold the tension briefly (the time may be gradually increased).

    C.   Relax thoroughly.

Repeat

Repeat the exercise a second time.

Ten Deep Breaths

After completing this entire series of tension/relaxation exercises, you will want to relax your muscles thoroughly. Remain lying in the corpse pose and take ten deep breaths. Pay special attention to the exhalations, exhaling fully. Do not allow any pause between breaths. Let the breath flow smoothly, without jerks and without sound. At the completion of these ten breaths you will feel refreshed and ready to continue.

PART THREE
The Boat Pose

34 / *Exercise Without Movement*

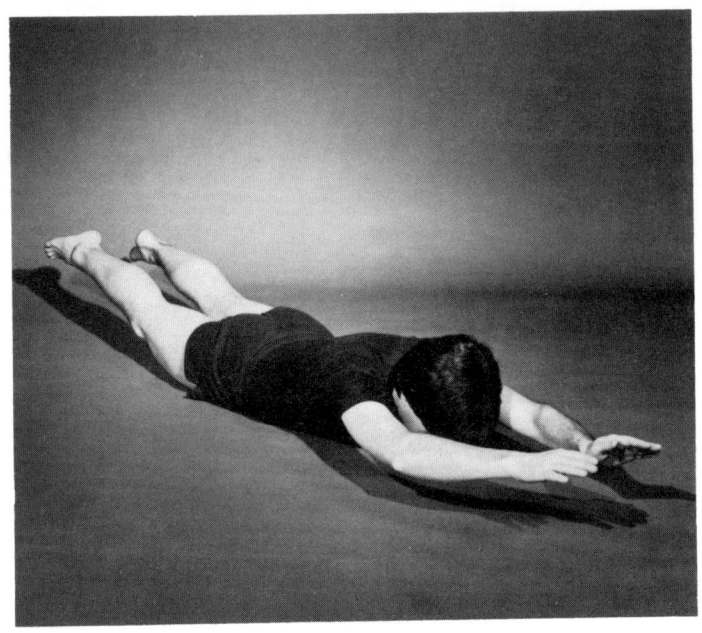

The boat pose

Boat Pose

Roll onto the stomach. With the feet about eighteen inches apart and the arms parallel, inhale and simultaneously raise the arms and the legs until only the stomach remains on the floor. The arms remain alongside the ears. The body forms a gentle curve from the tip of the toes to the fingers.

Hold for five seconds as you continue to breathe smoothly.

Exhaling, lower the body. Relax.

Note: You will find less tension in this posture if you allow the arms to be slightly lower than the legs. The weight of the body belongs at the navel.

Repeat

Practice the posture twice.

The boat posture is very beneficial. It strengthens all the muscles of the back. At the same time it increases intra-abdominal pressure and promotes better circulation to the internal organs.

Relaxed Breathing

Before going on to the next posture establish diaphragmatic breathing in the crocodile pose. Relax completely, giving special attention to relaxing the thighs and buttocks.

PART FOUR
Ashvini Mudra

38 / *Exercise Without Movement*

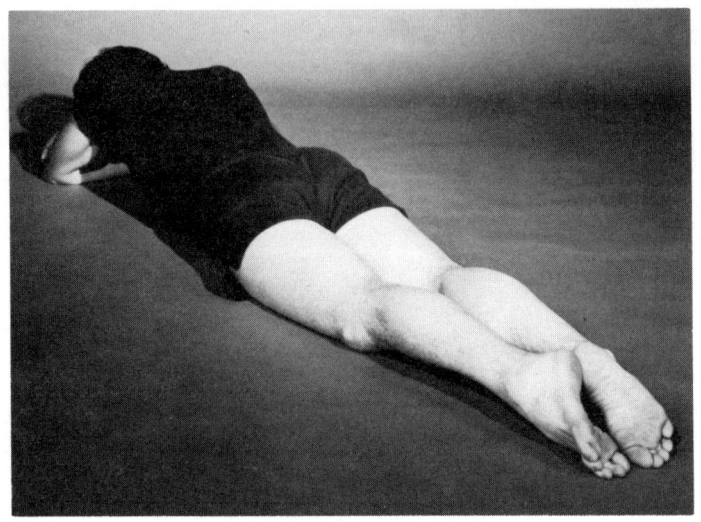

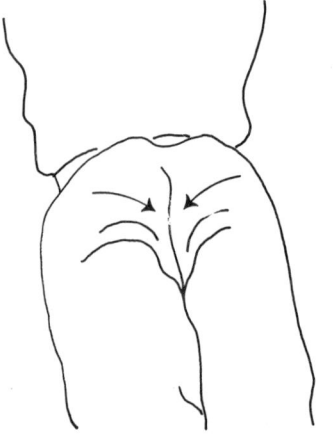

Ashvini mudra

Ashvini Mudra

This posture may be practiced either lying on the stomach or standing. Practice on the stomach until you have mastered the movements. After two or three weeks of practice, it may simply be included as part of the standing tension/relaxation, which will follow shortly.

Lie in the crocodile posture. Bring the legs together. Slowly roll the buttocks inward. Increase the tension, as if the anus is receding into the rectum. Tighten all the muscles inward, giving the effect of flattening the buttocks. The buttocks will be very firm. Hold briefly. Then slowly release the tension and relax.

Repeat

Perform the exercise a second time.

This posture tones the large buttock muscles. It is also applied in other yoga practices. Create the tension slowly, without jerks. At maximum tension, there will be a surface movement inward of up to nine or twelve inches.

Ten Deep Breaths

Complete the prone position exercises with ten deep breaths in the crocodile posture.

PART FIVE
The Child's Pose

42 / Exercise Without Movement

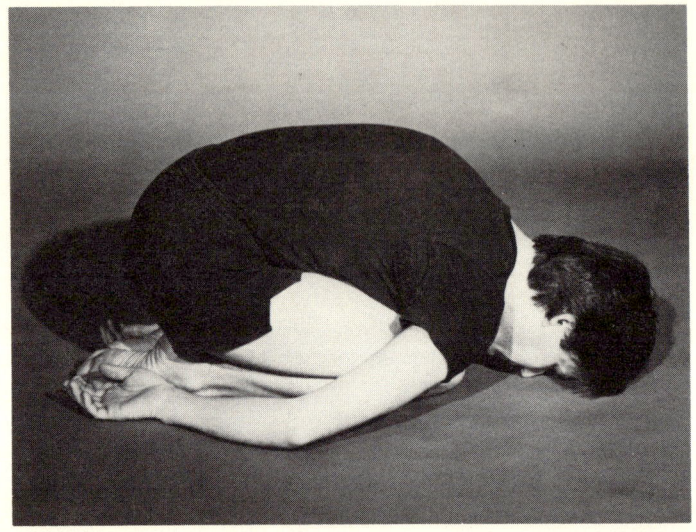

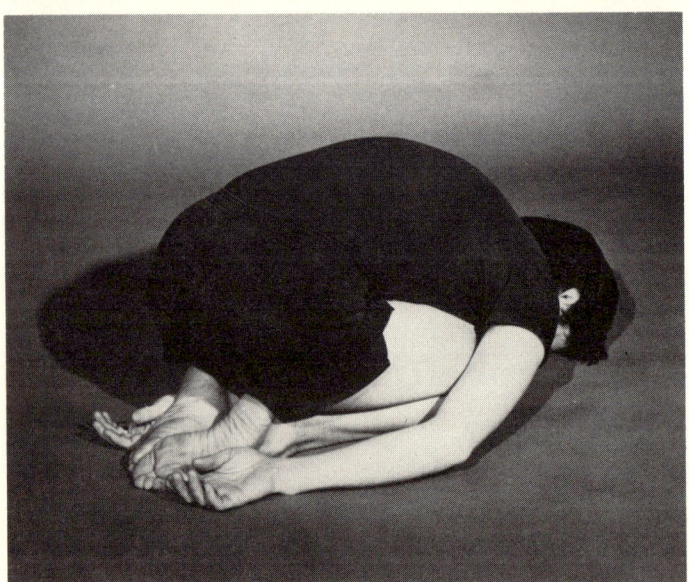

The child's pose

Child's Pose

The following exercise is not a tension/relaxation practice. The purpose of the exercise is to adjust and correctly place the intestines in their abdominal seat.

Assume the child's pose, as pictured, in the following way. Sit in a kneeling position with the top of the feet on the floor and the buttocks resting on the heels. Keep the head, neck, and trunk straight. Relax the arms, and rest the hands on the floor, with the palms upward and the fingers pointing behind you.

Exhaling, slowly bend forward from the hips until the stomach and chest rest on the thighs and the forehead touches the floor in front of the knees. As the body bends forward slide the hands back into a comfortable position.

Note: Do not lift the thighs or buttocks off the legs.

Breathe evenly. As you inhale you will feel the abdomen press against the thighs. Exhaling, the pressure is released.

Vigorous Breathing

Take five deep, vigorous breaths (five exhalations and inhalations) while holding the child's pose. Do not be concerned if there is noise or less control than usual. The abdomen should be vigorously drawn inward with the exhalation and fully expanded with the inhalation. After completing five breaths, slowly come back to a sitting posture on the heels. Let the circulation return to normal.

PART SIX
Standing Tension/Relaxation

46 / *Exercise Without Movement*

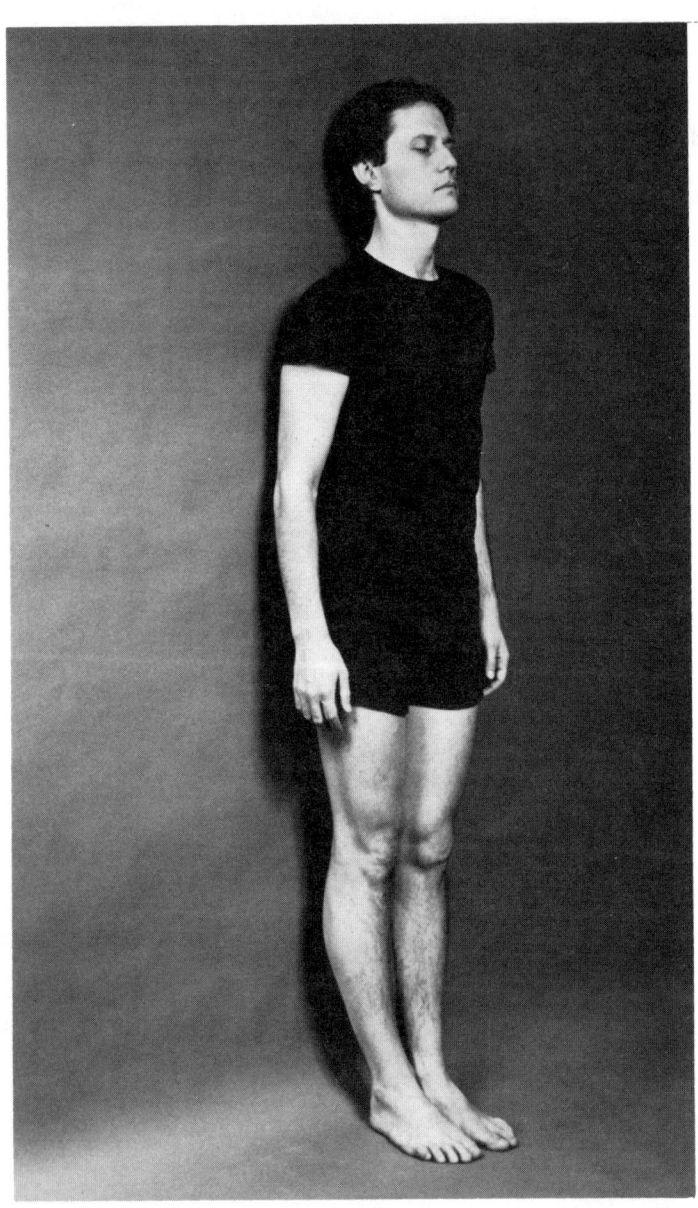

Standing against a wall

Standing Against a Wall

Stand erect with your body leaning against a wall. The heels will be a few inches from the wall and will be together. Allow the buttocks, shoulders, and head to rest against the wall. Without support, it is impossible to perform this exercise to perfection.

Relaxation: Head to Toe

While standing, relax slowly from the crown of the head down to the toes. (Specific muscle groups are listed in Appendix III.) After reaching the toes, breathe slowly twice.

Tension: Toe to Head

Tense the legs upward from toes to thighs. Perform ashvini mudra while maintaining the tension in the legs; then continue tensing upward along the joints of the spine. Tense each of the thirty-two vertebral joints, one by one, to the top of the spine and on to the crown of the head.

Hold the tension from the toes to the head. Hold only briefly at first, gradually increasing the time.

Relaxation: Toe to Head

Relax slowly and systematically from the toes to the crown, releasing all the tension.

Relaxed Breathing

Remain in the posture for a period of relaxed breathing.

Note: In this exercise, as the tension moves upward along the spine, the breath will become finer, with less volume of air being exchanged owing to peripheral tension in the abdomen and chest.

Repeat

Repeat the entire exercise.

PART SEVEN
Agni Sara

52 / *Exercise Without Movement*

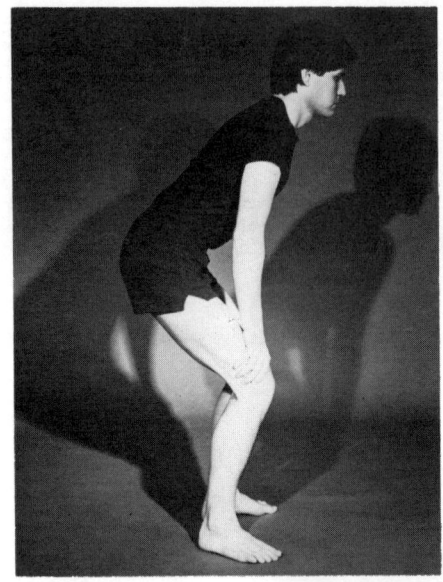

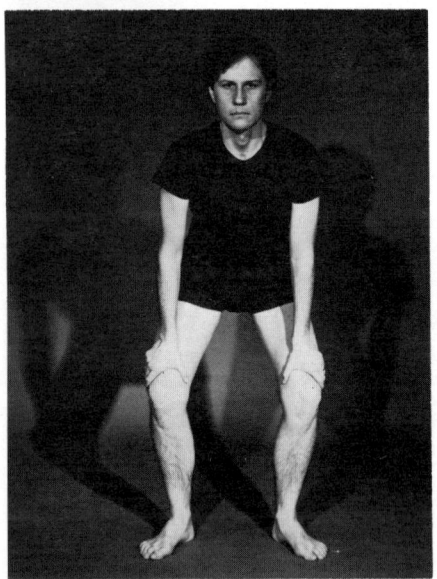

Agni sara

Agni Sara

Agni sara means "energizing the solar system," the area of the body associated with digestion. Agni sara also benefits the bowels, bladder, digestive system, nervous system, circulatory system, and reproductive system. Of all the exercises this one is the most beneficial, and if time is very short, it may be performed alone.

This exercise can be performed correctly only after discriminating between the abdominal and pelvic regions of the body. "Abdomen" is a general term for the large area extending from the diaphragm muscle down to the base of the trunk. The abdominal region is protected by two strong muscles, the abdominus rectus muscles. The lowest portion of the abdomen is more specifically called the "pelvis." The pelvis extends from a line slightly below the navel down to the pubic bone. The muscles of the pelvis may be contracted separately from the muscles in the higher navel and abdominal regions.

Note: It is for the above reason that the following exercise, agni sara, differs from the exercise commonly taught in beginning hatha yoga classes and given the same name. That exercise is actually a simple variation of the stomach lift and *will not* give the benefits described here.

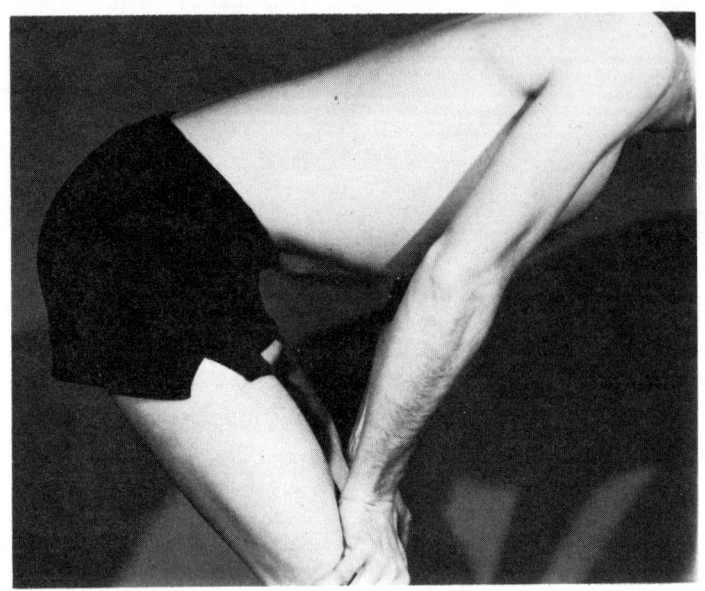

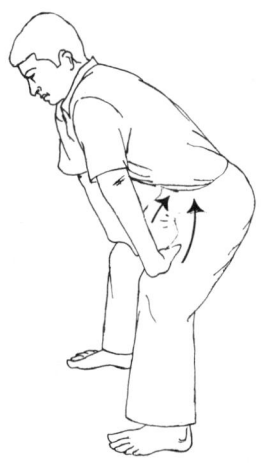

Pelvic contraction in agni sara

Practice

Assume the posture as pictured. The feet are comfortably apart, the knees bent, and the weight of the body rests on the arms. As you exhale, draw the *pelvic area* inward and up. Continue to contract this area as long as the exhalation continues. There is no retention of breath. As the inhalation begins, slowly release the contraction and let the pelvic muscles relax. Continue this systematic contraction and relaxation with each breath. If you tire or become short of breath, pause and breathe freely before continuing. Start with ten breaths. Gradually increase to as many as fifty breaths, or more.

It may take many months to acquire the control and stamina necessary to perform this exercise correctly. Do not become discouraged. Your efforts will be rewarded with excellent health.

PART EIGHT
Shavayatra

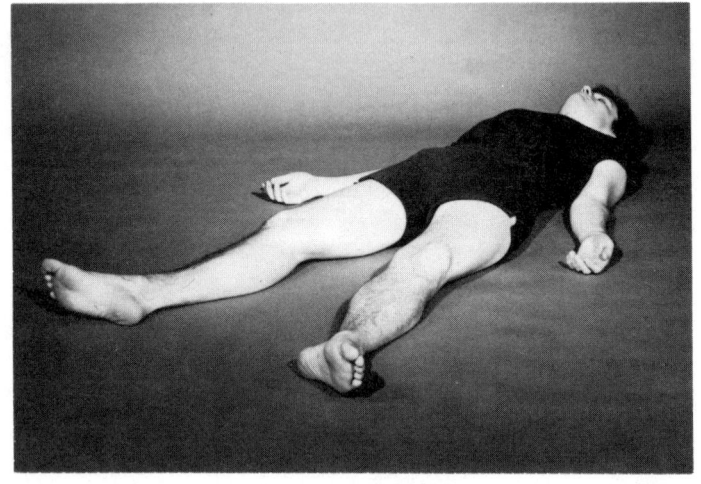

The corpse pose

Exercise Without Movement / 59

ONE
Relaxation

Lie on your back on a firm flat surface. The corpse pose relaxation practice is described in Appendix III and will be familiar to experienced students. After surveying and relaxing the whole body, go on to the exercise described below.

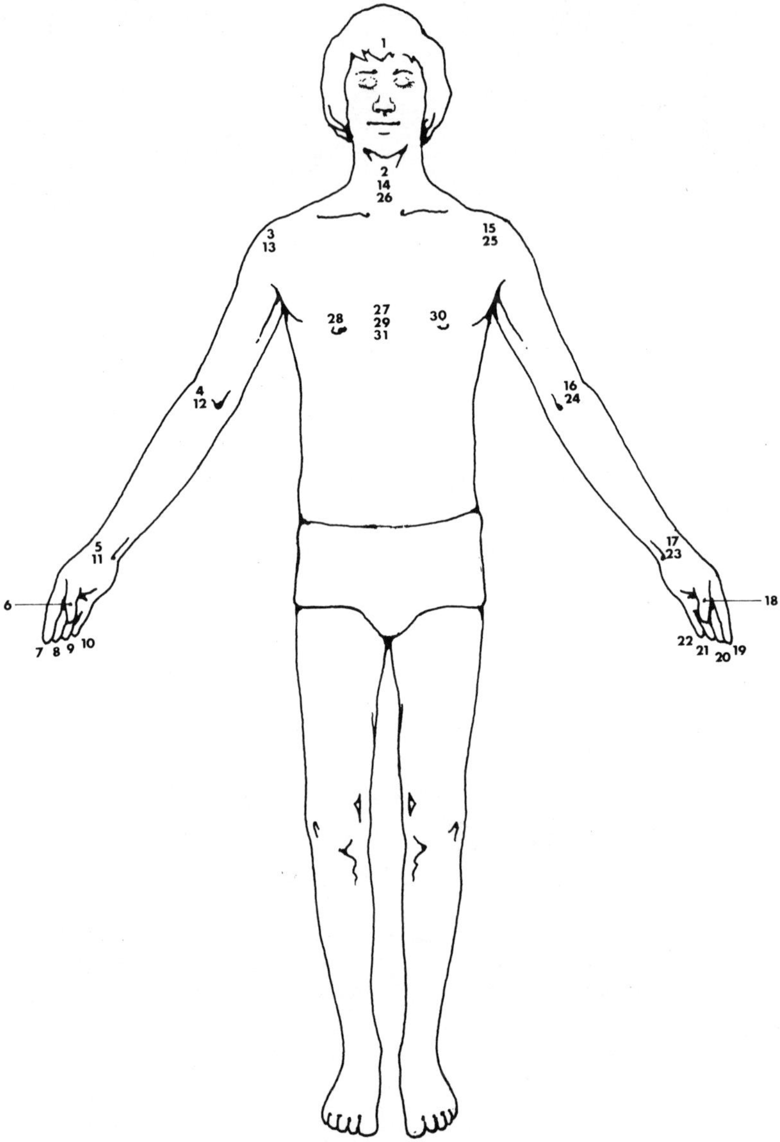
1
2
14
26
3
13
15
25
27
29
31
28
30
4
12
16
24
5
11
17
23
6
18
7 8 9 10
22 21 20 19

31 Points

TWO
31 Point Relaxation

In this exercise the mind is directed and focused on specific points of the body that help the student to survey weak or distressed areas. The mind closely inspects the body and can discover where problems lie. The order of progression is shown on the accompanying diagram.

Bring your attention to the point between the eyebrows and think the number "1." Keep the attention fixed at that point for one or two seconds. In the same manner continue concentrating on the numbered points through point 31, as pictured.

Repeat

Repeat the exercise from points 1 to 31 a second time. Practice in this way for seven to ten days.

Exercise Without Movement

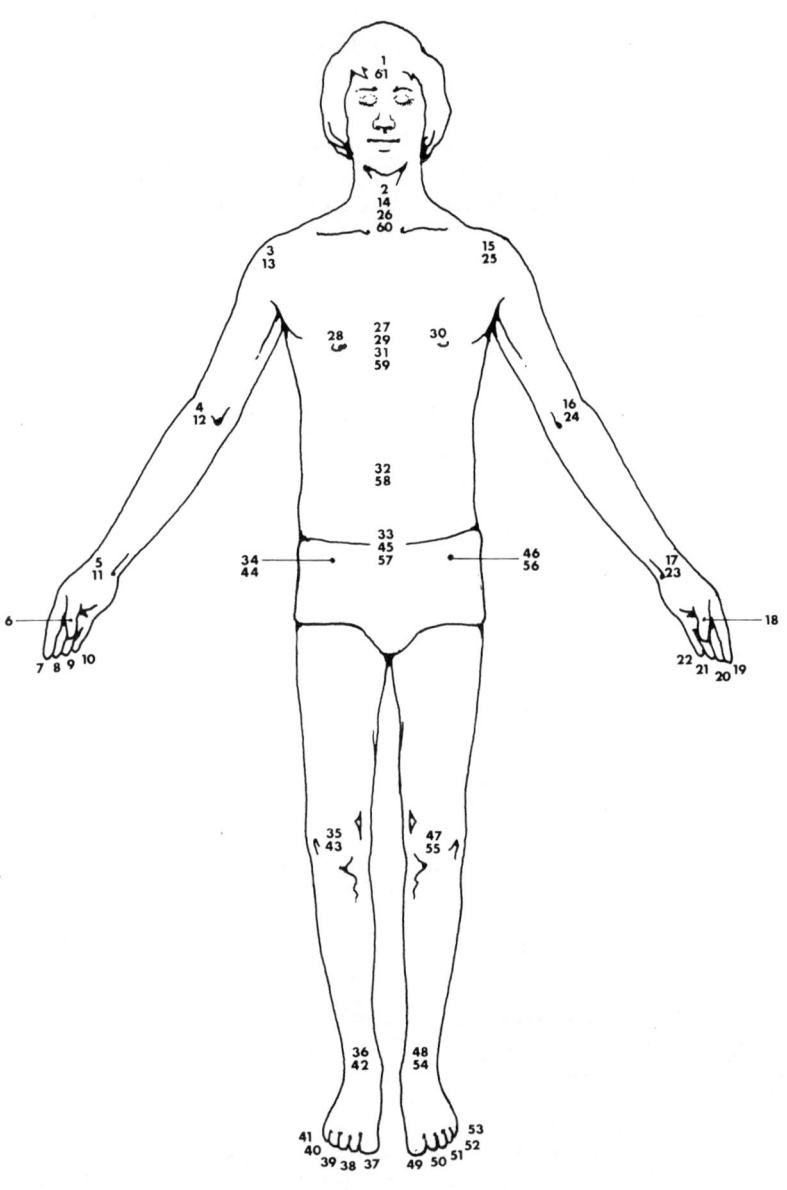

61 Points

THREE
61 Point Relaxation

When this exercise can be done without allowing the mind to wander, then continue through all the 61 points, as pictured. This exercise is called *shavayatra,* which means "inner traveling through the body."

FOUR
Ten Deep Relaxed Breaths

After completing the 61 point exercise, continue to lie in the corpse posture. Have the feeling that your body is lying on the sands of a warm tropical beach. With the exhalation imagine that a wave passes downward through the body, carrying away wastes, fatigue, and all worries. With the inhalation a fresh wave passes upward through the whole body, carrying a feeling of energy and well-being from an ocean of cosmic vitality. In this way breathe ten times. Then slowly open your eyes to the palms of your hands, let your attention come outward to the space around you, roll onto your side, and come back to a sitting posture.

PART NINE
Two to One Breathing

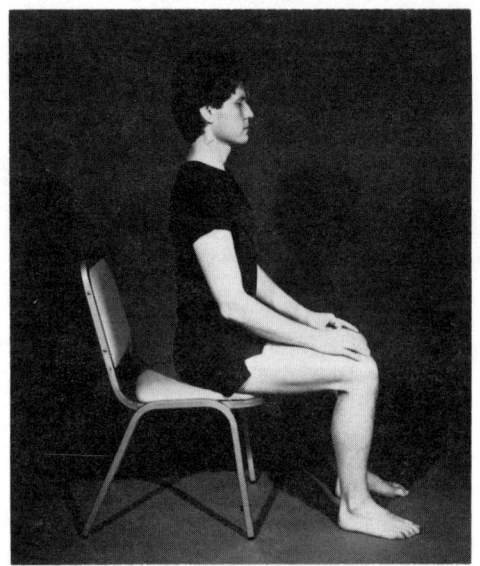

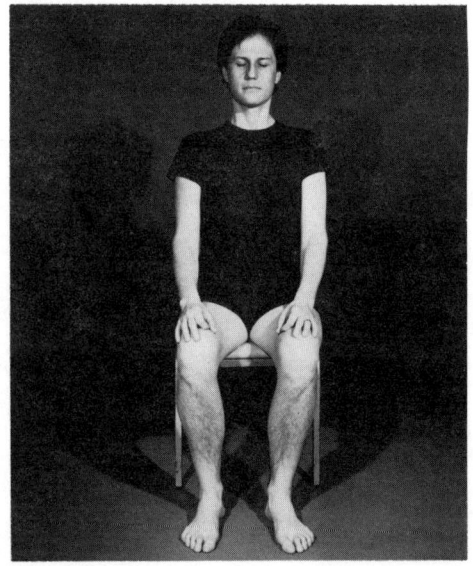

Sitting on a chair

Two to One Breathing

Sit with your head, neck, and trunk straight. Use a flat-seated chair or yoga meditation posture. Let your breath become deep and diaphragmatic, and again briefly survey your body, releasing any remaining tension.

Make your exhalation twice as long as the inhalation. In the beginning count in your mind six or eight for the exhalation, while counting three or four for the inhalation. Gradually the breath will become more fine and subtle, and the count will lengthen to sixteen (exhalation) and eight (inhalation), or more. The numbers are given as illustrations only, counting at about one count per second. Find the length of breath comfortable for you.

As this exercise continues, the pores of the body open, and the body brings forward waste matter to be expelled by the lungs. The mouth may become dry. The breath will become fine and serene.

68 / *Exercise Without Movement*

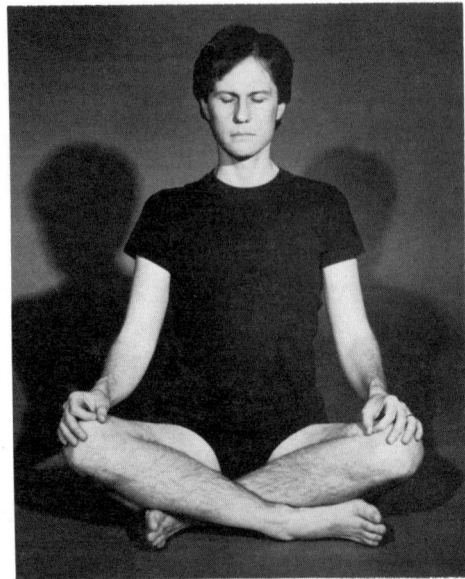

The easy pose

The auspicious pose

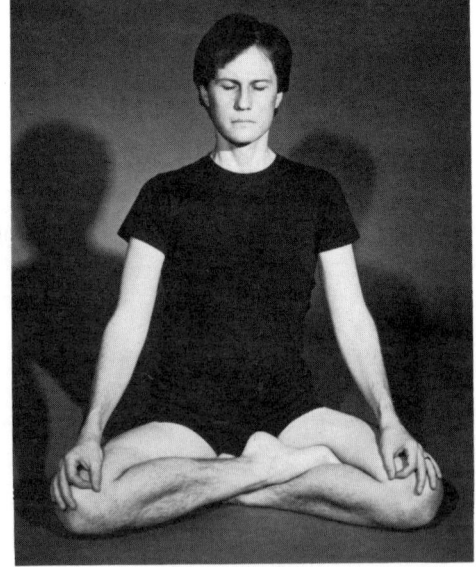

Begin with seven breaths, and increase gradually up to a period of three to five minutes. Experienced students may wish to continue with alternate nostril breathing (nadi shodana) and meditation.

Conclusion

The first stage of practice is now concluded. It may take many months to fully master all of the practices. Let the exercises become a part of your life and daily schedule. You will enjoy all the benefits that the exercises provide.

APPENDIX I
Preparations for Practice

The practice of hatha yoga is safe and beneficial. Some practical precautions insure the best results for every individual. Please read and observe the following:

1. Non-harming is the first principle of yoga. Do not harm your body or mind by exceeding your capacity and thereby allowing mental tension to become associated with your practice.

2. There is no competition in yoga. Be comfortable and mentally content, but do not be lazy.

3. Wait three to four hours after meals and one-half hour after liquids before beginning practice.

4. Empty the bladder before practicing and train the bowels to be regular.

5. If current or recent medical problems exist, consult with your physician before beginning practice.

6. During a woman's menstruation, the relaxation and breathing exercises are very beneficial, but the other exercises should not be practiced until the body has completed its natural cleansing.

7. Use common sense in all yoga practices. Care for your body, breath, and mind.

Many publications of the Himalayan International Institute, available throughout the world, can assist the student in fully understanding the means and goals of yoga practice. Please examine the complete list of publications in the back of this manual for more information.

APPENDIX II
Diaphragmatic Breathing

The diaphragm is a muscle that divides the torso into two separate chambers, the thorax and the abdomen. The diaphragm forms the floor of the thorax, and rests against the base of the lungs. As it relaxes, this dome-shaped muscle presses against the lungs from below, causing exhalation. Inhalation follows as the diaphragm contracts. In a healthy person this alternating movement of the diaphragm is responsible for seventy-five percent of the exchange of gases in the lungs. Commonly, however, the diaphragm is abnormally tense, and natural breathing is blocked altogether. This results in symptoms of fatigue, underlying tension, and even more serious problems. One of the first aims of yoga is to re-establish good breathing habits, thus improving both physical and mental health.

Feel the correct movement of diaphragmatic breathing by lying in the crocodile posture as illustrated at the beginning of this manual. The diaphragm moves vertically in the body, pressing against the lungs from below. Signs of correct diaphragmatic breathing can easily be observed

74 / *Exercise Without Movement*

in the crocodile pose. Inhaling, the abdomen expands, pressing against the floor below. Exhaling, the abdomen contracts. Similarly, when inhaling, the back gently rises, and when exhaling, it gently falls. Both these effects are produced by correct movement of the diaphragm.

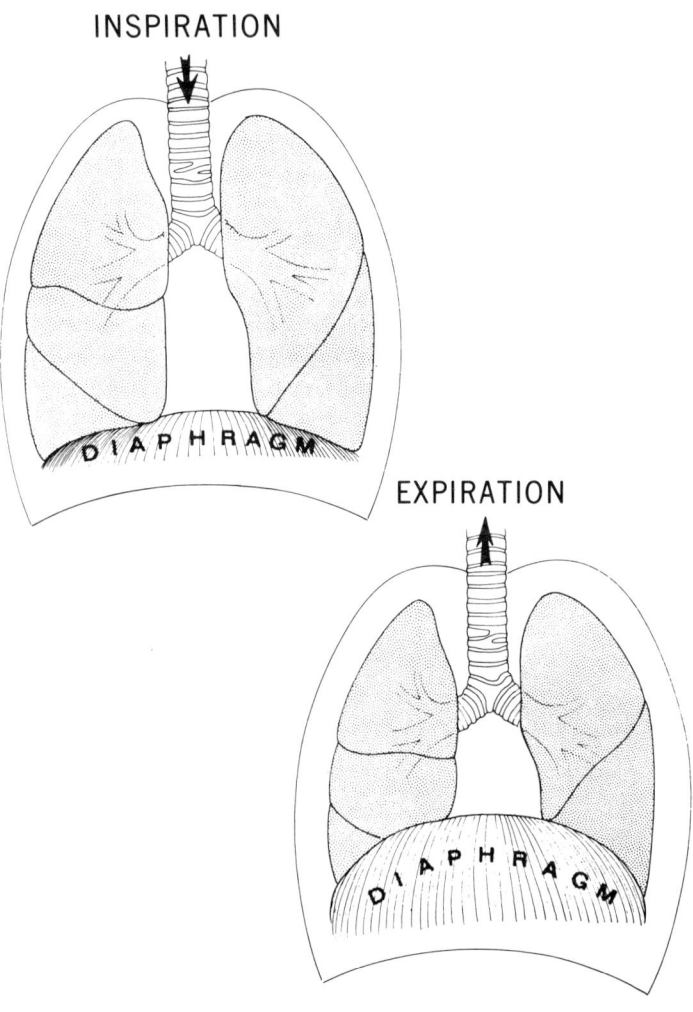

The diaphragm

Establish the habit of diaphragmatic breathing in daily life—twenty-four hours a day. It does not take long. Practice the crocodile pose three times daily for five to ten minutes each time. When finished, roll onto the back briefly, relaxing and observing the breath. In this posture the abdomen will continue to expand and contract. Next, sit up in a chair and again watch the breathing process, relaxing the abdomen. Finally, stand as you continue to breathe diaphragmatically. Practice regularly until diaphragmatic breathing is established.

The following criteria will help to evaluate the breathing process:

1. The breath flows smoothly, without jerks.

2. There is no pause between the breaths.

3. The breath flows silently in the lungs and air passageways.

4. Exhalation and inhalation are approximately equal.

5. The breath is deep, yet there is little movement of the upper chest.

Diaphragmatic breathing enables you to feel your best, gain emotional control and balance, and reduce fatigue and stress. The habit of diaphragmatic breathing is required for all other yoga breathing practices.

76 / *Exercise Without Movement*

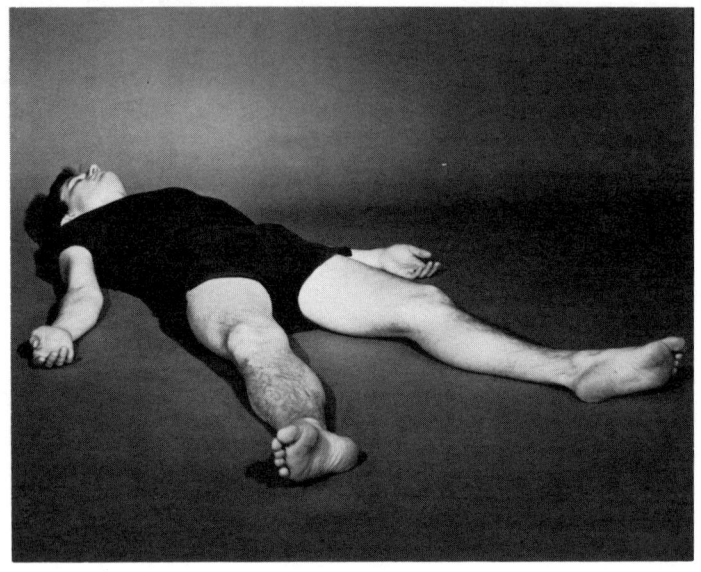

The corpse pose

APPENDIX III
Corpse Pose Relaxation

The word "relaxation" may be somewhat misleading. If one "tries" to relax, the effort is bound to fail. Nor by repeating the word "relax, relax" is much progress made. Relaxation must be learned systematically and then allowed to progress naturally. In relaxation one learns the art of letting go.

There are many methods of yoga relaxation. The following exercise forms the base from which many succeeding exercises may be learned. It is effective in relieving tension and helps to bring the mind into a state of relaxed concentration.

Practice

Lie on your back in the corpse pose as illustrated at the beginning of this manual. Use a thin cushion under the head. Cover your body with a sheet or thin shawl. Place the legs a comfortable distance apart. The arms are slightly separated from the body, and the palms are turned up. Most important, the spine should not be bent to either side. Take time to adjust your posture and then become still.

Closing your eyes, become aware of the presence of your body, the spaces around you, and the place on which your body rests. Observe the whole body from head to toes. Cultivate and enjoy the stillness of your body—perfect stillness, except for the slow and gentle movement of your breathing.

Now bring your attention to your breath. Observe each exhalation and inhalation, and let the breath become deep and diaphragmatic. Breathing out, release all your tension, waste, fatigue, and worry. Inhale a feeling of energy and well-being. Do not pause between the breaths.

Now gently survey your body mentally. At the places of observation where there is tension, you will naturally release it. This process of "letting go" is the relaxation process. Proceed from the head to the toes, and then back to the head, following the sequence indicated below.

    forehead
    eyebrows and eyes
    nose*

    cheeks
    mouth
    jaw
    chin
    neck
    shoulders
    upper arms
    lower arms
    hands
    fingers
    fingertips*

fingers
hands
lower arms
upper arms
shoulders
chest
heart center**

stomach
navel region
pelvic region
upper legs
lower legs
feet
toes**

Now reverse the order and proceed upward, this time without any pauses.

At these places, as you proceed from the head to the toes, you may pause for two or four** relaxed breaths. There are no pauses for breathing as you proceed upward from toes to head.

Some practice will be required to complete this exercise without losing attention. If the mind wanders, simply and gently bring it back to the relaxation process.

After progressing through the whole body, gently relax your mind. Turn your attention to the quiet flow of your breathing, and observe the entire breathing process. For a few minutes, lie resting, feeling that this subtle stream of breath is a link joining you to the cosmos. You will be in harmony and at peace. After resting briefly, once more roll to your side and sit up.

APPENDIX IV
Summary at a Glance

PART ONE
Basic Relaxation

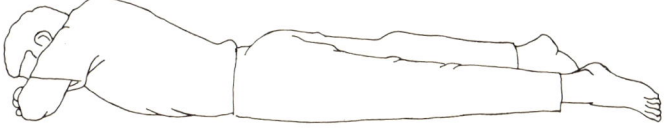

Crocodile Relaxation

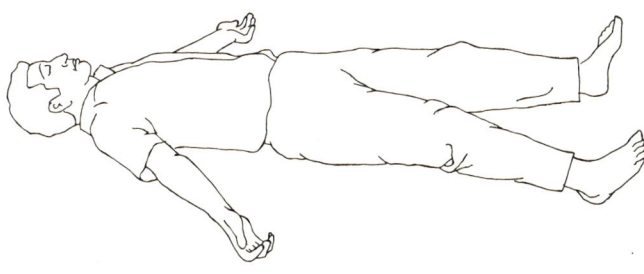

Corpse Relaxation

82 / *Exercise Without Movement*

PART TWO
Tension/Relaxation Exercise

ONE

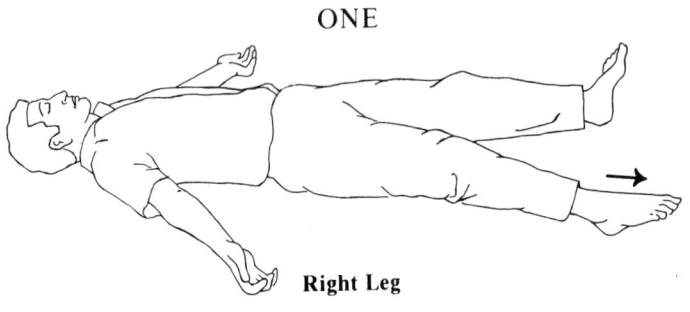

Right Leg

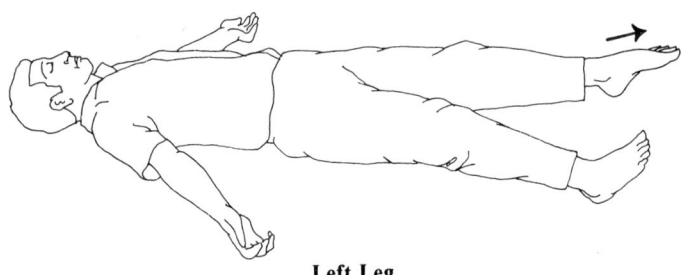

Left Leg

Repeat

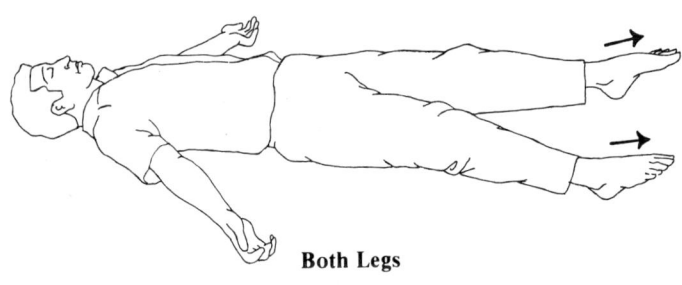

Both Legs
Repeat
Relaxed Breathing

TWO

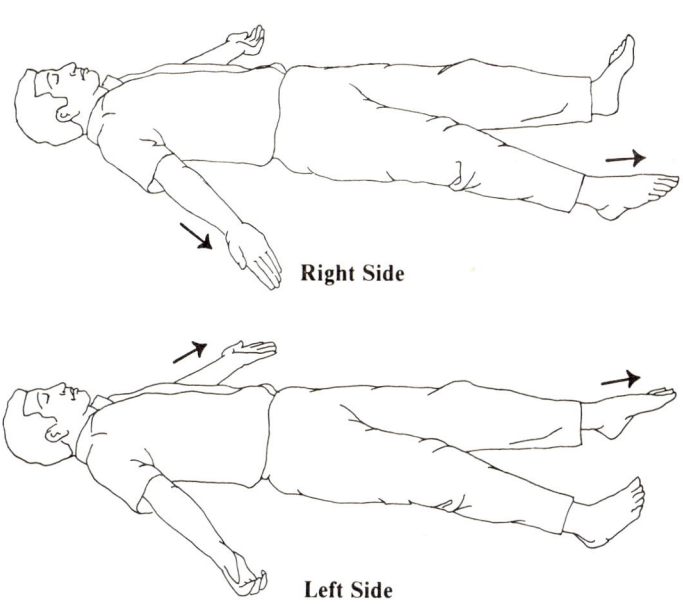

Repeat
Relaxed Breathing

THREE

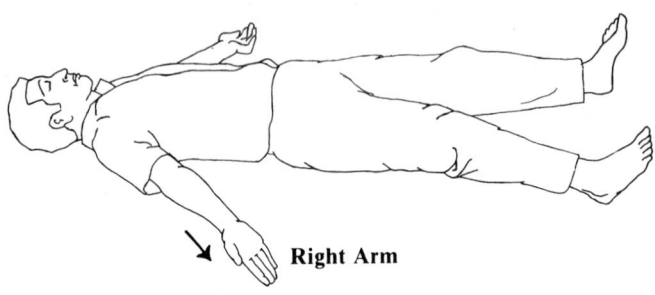

Right Arm

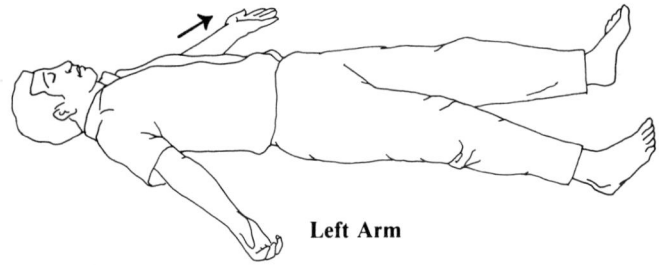

Left Arm

Repeat

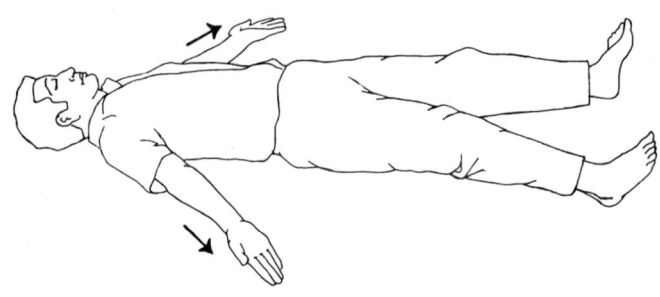

Both Arms
Repeat
Relaxed Breathing

FOUR

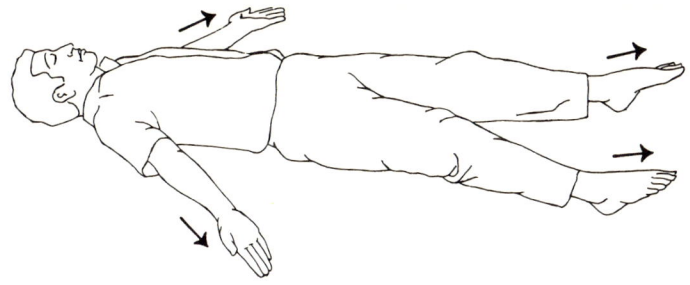

All Limbs
Repeat
Ten Deep Breaths

PART THREE
The Boat Pose

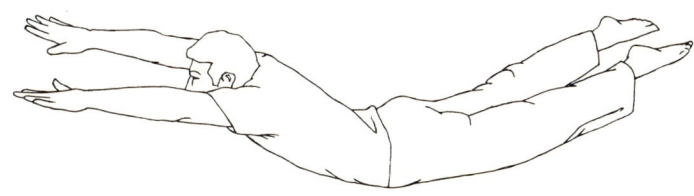

The Boat Pose
Repeat
Relaxed Breathing

86 / *Exercise Without Movement*

PART FOUR
Ashvini Mudra

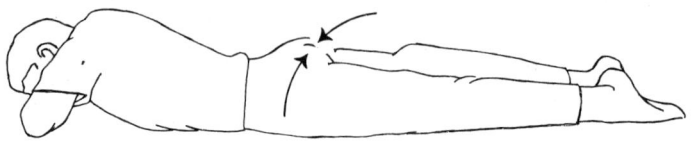

Ashvini Mudra
Repeat
Ten Deep Breaths

PART FIVE
The Child's Pose

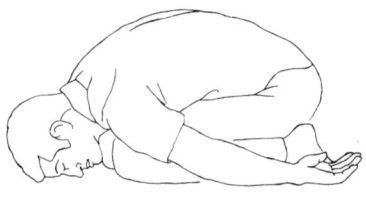

The Child's Pose
Five Vigorous Breaths

Exercise Without Movement / 87

PART SIX
Standing Tension/Relaxation

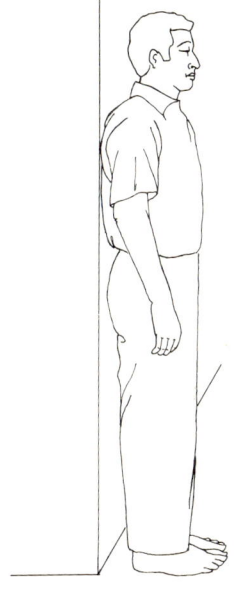

Relax Head to Toe
Tense Toe to Head
Relax Toe to Head
Relaxed Breathing
Repeat

PART SEVEN
Agni Sara

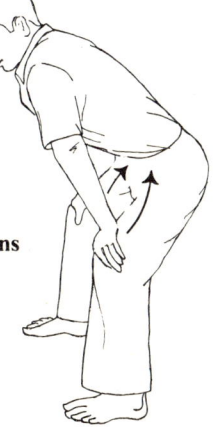

Agni Sara
Ten to Fifty Pelvic Contractions

PART EIGHT
Shavayatra

Relaxation
31 Points (twice)
or 61 Points
Ten Deep Relaxed Breaths

PART NINE
Two to One Breathing

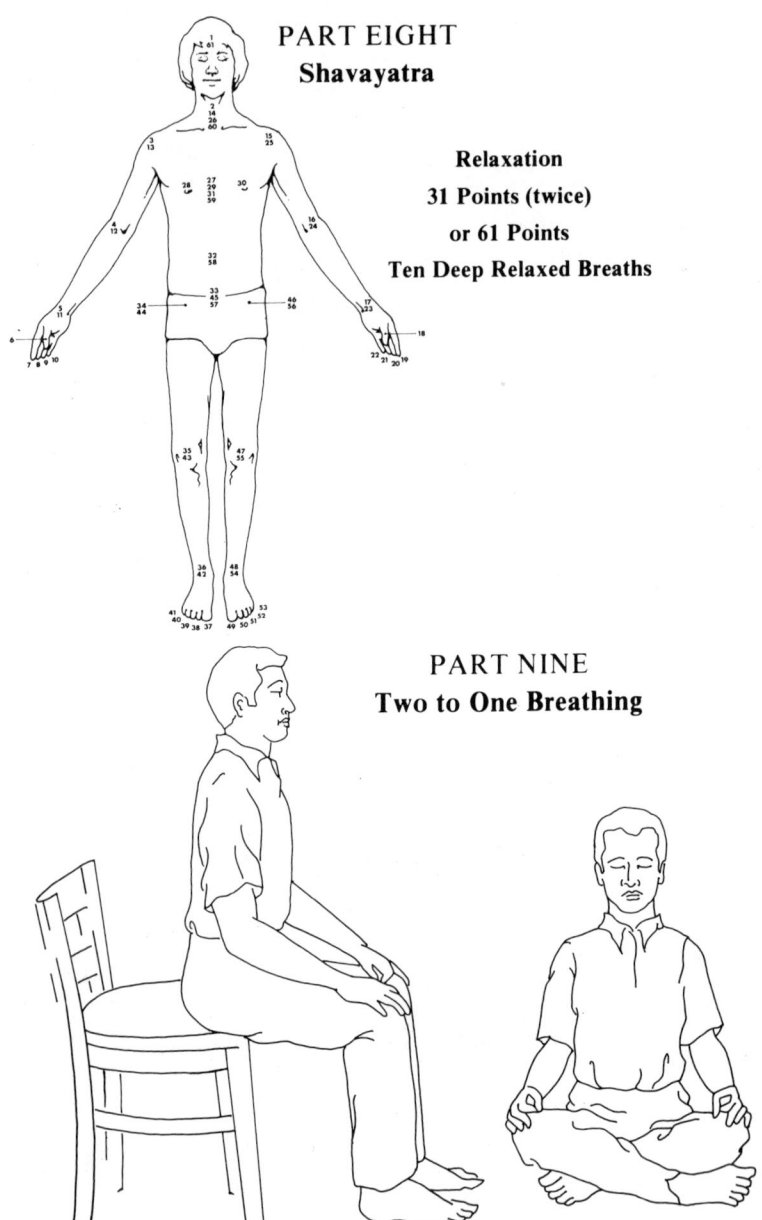

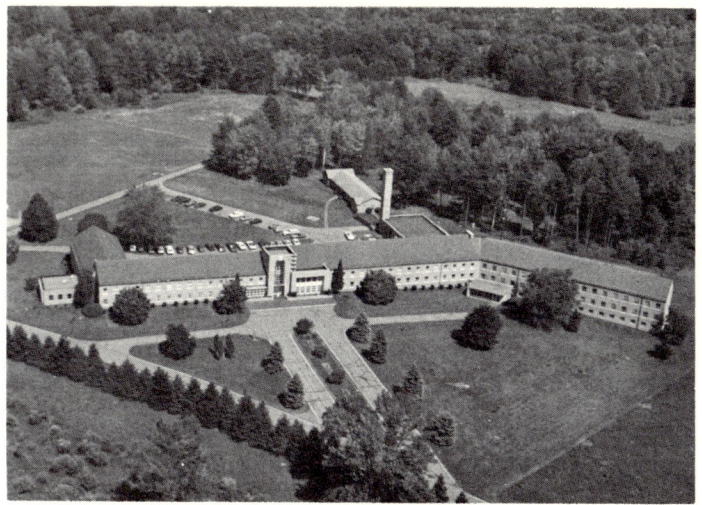

The main building of the national headquarters, Honesdale, Pa.

The Himalayan Institute

The Himalayan International Institute of Yoga Science and Philosophy of the U.S.A. is a nonprofit organization devoted to the scientific and spiritual progress of modern humanity. Founded in 1971 by Sri Swami Rama, the Institute combines Western and Eastern teachings and techniques to develop educational, therapeutic, and research programs for serving people in today's world. The goals of the Institute are to teach meditational techniques for the growth of individuals and their society, to make known the harmonious view of world religions and philosophies, and to undertake scientific research for the benefit of humankind.

This challenging task is met by people of all ages, all walks of life, and all faiths who attend and participate in the Institute courses and seminars. These programs, which are given on a continuing basis, are designed in order that one may discover for oneself how to live more creatively. In the words of Swami Rama, "By being aware of one's own potential and abilities, one can become a perfect citizen, help the nation, and serve humanity."

The Institute has branch centers and affiliates throughout the United States. The 422-acre campus of the national headquarters, located in the Pocono Mountains of northeastern Pennsylvania, serves as the coordination center for all the Institute activities, which include a wide variety of innovative programs in education, research, and therapy, combining Eastern and Western approaches to self-awareness and self-directed change.

SEMINARS, LECTURES, WORKSHOPS, and CLASSES are available throughout the year, providing intensive training and experience in such topics as Superconscious Meditation, hatha yoga, philosophy, psychology, and various aspects of personal growth and holistic health. The *Himalayan News*, a free bimonthly publication, announces the current programs.

The RESIDENTIAL and SELF-TRANSFORMATION PROGRAMS provide training in the basic yoga disciplines—diet, ethical behavior, hatha yoga, and meditation. Students are also given guidance in a philosophy of living in a community environment.

The PROGRAM IN EASTERN STUDIES AND COMPARATIVE PSYCHOLOGY is a program of academic study for post-baccalaureate students that offers a systematic synthesis of Western empirical sciences with Eastern introspective sciences using both practical and traditional approaches to education. Course work from the Program in Eastern Studies may be applied toward individually designed Master's and Doctoral degrees obtained from several accredited colleges and universities.

The five-day STRESS MANAGEMENT PROGRAM offers practical and individualized training that can be used to control the stress response. This includes biofeedback, relaxation skills, exercise, diet, breathing techniques, and meditation.

A yearly INTERNATIONAL CONGRESS, sponsored by the Institute, is devoted to the scientific and spiritual progress of modern humanity. Through lectures, workshops, seminars, and practical demonstrations, it provides a forum for professionals and lay people to share their knowledge and research.

The ELEANOR N. DANA RESEARCH LABORATORY is the psychophysiological laboratory of the Institute, specializing in research on breathing, meditation, holistic therapies, and stress and relaxed states. The laboratory is fully equipped for exercise stress testing and psychophysiological measurements, including brain waves, patterns of respiration, heart rate changes, and muscle tension. The staff investigates Eastern teachings through studies based on Western experimental techniques.

Himalayan Institute Publications

Living with the Himalayan Masters	Swami Rama
Lectures on Yoga	Swami Rama
A Practical Guide to Holistic Health	Swami Rama
Choosing a Path	Swami Rama
Inspired Thoughts of Swami Rama	Swami Rama
Freedom from the Bondage of Karma	Swami Rama
Book of Wisdom (Ishopanishad)	Swami Rama
Enlightenment Without God	Swami Rama
Exercise Without Movement	Swami Rama
Life Here and Hereafter	Swami Rama
Marriage, Parenthood, and Enlightenment	Swami Rama
Path of Fire and Light	Swami Rama
Perennial Psychology of the Bhagavad Gita	Swami Rama
Love Whispers	Swami Rama
Celestial Song/Gobind Geet	Swami Rama
Creative Use of Emotion	Swami Rama, Swami Ajaya
Science of Breath	Swami Rama, Rudolph Ballentine, M.D., Alan Hymes, M.D.
Yoga and Psychotherapy	Swami Rama, Rudolph Ballentine, M.D., Swami Ajaya
Yoga-sutras of Patanjali	Usharbudh Arya, D.Litt.
Superconscious Meditation	Usharbudh Arya, D.Litt.
Mantra and Meditation	Usharbudh Arya, D.Litt.
Philosophy of Hatha Yoga	Usharbudh Arya, D.Litt.
Meditation and the Art of Dying	Usharbudh Arya, D.Litt.
God	Usharbudh Arya, D.Litt.
Psychotherapy East and West: A Unifying Paradigm	Swami Ajaya, Ph.D.
Yoga Psychology	Swami Ajaya, Ph.D.
Psychology East and West	Swami Ajaya, Ph.D. (ed.)

Meditational Therapy	Swami Ajaya, Ph.D. (ed.)
Diet and Nutrition	Rudolph Ballentine, M.D.
Joints and Glands Exercises	Rudolph Ballentine, M.D. (ed.)
Theory and Practice of Meditation	Rudolph Ballentine, M.D. (ed.)
Freedom from Stress	Phil Nuernberger, Ph.D.
Science Studies Yoga	James Funderburk, Ph.D.
Homeopathic Remedies	Drs. Anderson, Buegel, Chernin
Hatha Yoga Manual I	Samskrti and Veda
Hatha Yoga Manual II	Samskrti and Judith Franks
Seven Systems of Indian Philosophy	R. Tigunait, Ph.D.
Swami Rama of the Himalayas	L. K. Misra, Ph.D. (ed.)
Philosophy of Death and Dying	M. V. Kamath
Practical Vedanta of Swami Rama Tirtha	Brandt Dayton (ed.)
The Swami and Sam	Brandt Dayton
Yoga and Christianity	Justin O'Brien, D.Th.
Himalayan Mountain Cookery	Martha Ballentine
The Yoga Way Cookbook	Himalayan Institute
Meditation in Christianity	Himalayan Institute
Art and Science of Meditation	Himalayan Institute
Therapeutic Value of Yoga	Himalayan Institute
Chants from Eternity	Himalayan Institute
Spiritual Diary	Himalayan Institute
Blank Books	Himalayan Institute

Write for a free mail order catalog describing all our publications.